LIVER CARE DOG FOOD

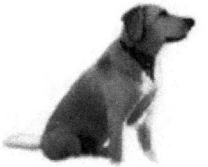

Brian L. Ayala

Copyright © 2024 by **Brian L. Ayala**

All rights reserved. No part of this book may be reproduced or transmitted in any form or by any means, electronic or mechanical, including photocopying, recording, or by any information storage and retrieval system, without permission in writing from the publisher.

TABLE OF CONTENTS

CHAPTER 1: 5
UNDERSTANDING CANINE LIVER HEALTH 5
- ❖ The Importance of the Liver in Dogs 5
- ❖ Common Liver Issues in Dogs (e.g., liver disease, toxicity, failure) 9
- ❖ Signs and Symptoms of Liver Problems in Dogs (e.g., vomiting, diarrhea, lethargy) 13

CHAPTER 2: 17
NUTRITION AND LIVER HEALTH 17
- ❖ The Role of Diet in Supporting Liver Function 17
- ❖ Key Nutrients for Liver Health (e.g., vitamin E, omega-3 fatty acids, antioxidants) 21
- ❖ How Hill's Prescription Diet l/d Supports Liver Health 25

CHAPTER 3: 29
HILL'S PRESCRIPTION DIET L/D LIVER CARE DOG FOOD 29
- ❖ Overview of the Product and its Formulation 29
- ❖ Key Ingredients and Their Benefits (e.g., high-quality protein, fiber, essential vitamins and minerals) 33
- ❖ Feeding Guidelines and Transitioning to the Diet 38

CHAPTER 4: 43
MANAGING LIVER DISEASE IN DOGS 43
- ❖ Diagnosis and Treatment Options (e.g., medication, surgery, dietary changes) 43
- ❖ Supporting Your Dog's Recovery and Ongoing Care 48
- ❖ Monitoring Progress and Adjusting the Diet as Needed 53

CHAPTER 5: 58
PREVENTING LIVER ISSUES AND PROMOTING OVERALL HEALTH 58
- ❖ Tips for Maintaining a Healthy Liver 58
- ❖ The Importance of Regular Veterinary Check-Ups and Monitoring 63
- ❖ A Holistic Approach to Supporting Your Dog's Overall Health and Wellbeing, 68

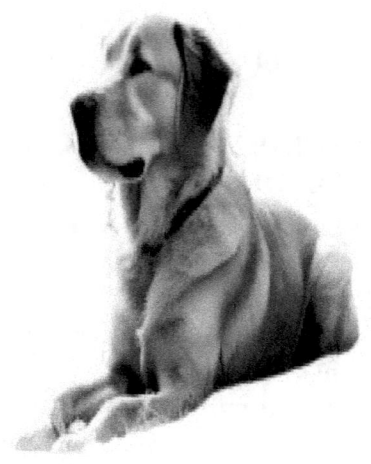

CHAPTER 1: UNDERSTANDING CANINE LIVER HEALTH

The Importance of the Liver in Dogs

The liver stands as one of the most vital organs in a dog's body, performing a multitude of essential functions that are crucial for their overall health and well-being. Often described as the body's chemical factory, the liver is responsible for a wide array of metabolic processes, detoxification, and nutrient storage. Understanding the pivotal role of the liver in canine health is paramount for ensuring the longevity and vitality of our beloved furry companions.

1. **Metabolism and Digestion**: The liver plays a central role in metabolism, breaking down nutrients from food into substances that can be utilized by the body. Carbohydrates, fats, and proteins are processed and converted into energy sources or stored for later use. For instance, the liver helps regulate blood sugar levels by storing excess glucose as glycogen and releasing it when needed to maintain a steady supply of energy. Any disruption in these metabolic functions can lead to various health issues such as diabetes or obesity in dogs.

2. **Detoxification**: One of the liver's primary functions is detoxification, filtering harmful toxins and waste products from the bloodstream. Dogs are constantly exposed to toxins from various sources including environmental pollutants, medications, and even certain foods. The liver neutralizes these toxins, making them less harmful and facilitating their excretion from the body. Without efficient detoxification, dogs can suffer from liver damage, leading to serious health complications.

3. **Production of Bile**: The liver produces bile, a digestive fluid that aids in the breakdown and absorption of fats in the intestine. Bile is essential for the digestion and utilization of dietary fats, as well as the elimination of waste products from the body. Any impairment in bile production can result in digestive issues such as fat malabsorption and nutrient deficiencies.

4. **Storage of Vitamins and Minerals**: The liver serves as a storage reservoir for various vitamins and minerals, including vitamin A, vitamin D, vitamin B12, and iron. These nutrients are essential for maintaining the dog's overall health and supporting vital functions such as immune system function, bone health, and red blood cell production. A healthy liver ensures proper storage

and utilization of these nutrients, preventing deficiencies and associated health problems.

5. **Synthesis of Proteins**: The liver synthesizes proteins that are necessary for blood clotting, immune function, and maintaining fluid balance within the body. Albumin, for example, is a protein produced by the liver that helps maintain blood volume and pressure. Dogs with liver disease may experience decreased synthesis of these proteins, leading to clotting disorders, weakened immune response, and edema.

Case Study: Canine Hepatic Disease

Consider the case of Max, a 7-year-old Labrador Retriever, who presented with symptoms of lethargy, decreased appetite, and vomiting. Upon examination, Max was diagnosed with hepatic disease, a condition characterized by inflammation or damage to the liver tissue. Further tests revealed elevated liver enzymes and impaired liver function.

Max's hepatic disease was attributed to various factors including exposure to toxic substances, underlying infections, and poor dietary habits. The dysfunction of his liver compromised its ability to perform essential functions such as detoxification, metabolism, and bile production. Without prompt intervention and proper management, Max's condition could have progressed to liver failure, posing a grave risk to his health and well-being.

The liver plays a pivotal role in maintaining the overall health and vitality of dogs, performing essential functions that are indispensable for their survival. From metabolism and detoxification to digestion and nutrient storage, the liver influences virtually every aspect of a dog's physiology. Understanding the importance of liver health and taking proactive measures to support it through proper nutrition, regular veterinary care, and the avoidance of toxins are crucial for ensuring the longevity and well-being of our canine companions.

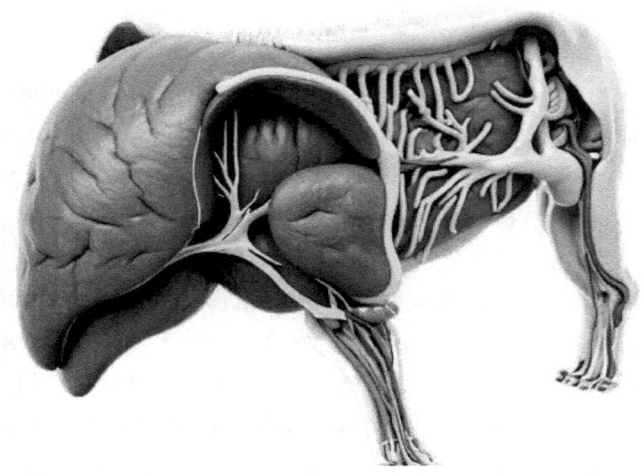

An illustration or diagram of the canine liver and its location in the body

Common Liver Issues in Dogs (e.g., liver disease, toxicity, failure)

When it comes to the body of a dog, the liver is an essential organ; yet, it is sadly prone to a variety of health problems that may have an impact on both its form and its function. For early identification, rapid treatment, and efficient management of these disorders, it is essential to have a solid understanding of the frequent liver problems that dogs may potentially have.

It is important to note that the term "liver disease" refers to a wide range of disorders that have an impact on the structure and function of the liver in dogs. Hepatitis, which is an inflammation of the liver, cirrhosis, which is scarring of the liver tissue, and hepatic lipidosis, which is an accumulation of fat in the liver cells, are some of the conditions that may be present. Several factors, including infectious agents, toxins, genetic predispositions, and underlying health disorders like diabetes or Cushing's syndrome, may all contribute to the development of liver disease. There is a wide range of symptoms that may be associated with liver illness in dogs; however, the most common ones include lethargy, reduced appetite, vomiting, diarrhea, jaundice (yellowing of the skin and eyes), and diarrhea. Intervention and diagnosis at an early stage are very necessary for the management of liver disease and the prevention of its development tintomore severe phases.

2. **Poisoning:** Dogs are vulnerable to liver poisoning as a result of exposure to a wide variety of substances, including some drugs, chemicals found in the home, plants, and components found in food. For example, intake of human drugs like acetaminophen (Tylenol) or xylitol (a sugar replacement) may induce liver damage in dogs. Similarly, eating some plants such as sago palm or ingestion of hazardous foods like grapes, raisins, or onions may lead to liver poisoning. Symptoms of liver poisoning may include vomiting, diarrhea, stomach discomfort, jaundice, convulsions, and coma. Prompt veterinary care is necessary if poisoning is suspected, since prompt treatment may help avoid irreparable liver damage and improve the prognosis.

3. **Liver Failure**: Liver failure happens when the liver is no longer able to conduct its vital tasks efficiently. It might come from acute liver damage, chronic liver disease, or underlying health issues that affect liver function. Liver failure may be classed as acute or chronic, based on the onset and course of symptoms. Acute liver failure is characterized by a quick onset of severe symptoms, typically needing emergency medical intervention. Chronic liver failure, on the other hand, develops

gradually over time, with symptoms deteriorating steadily. Common indications of liver failure in dogs include jaundice, fluid collection in the belly (ascites), neurological problems, and bleeding issues. Treatment of liver failure may require supportive care, dietary control, medicines to promote liver function, and, in extreme situations, liver transplantation.

Case Study: Canine Liver Disease Due to Toxin Exposure

Meet Bella, a 4-year-old Yorkshire Terrier who was taken to the veterinary clinic with symptoms of vomiting, lethargy, and jaundice. Upon investigation, Bella's liver enzymes were discovered to be considerably increased, suggesting liver dysfunction. After further investigation, it was determined that Bella had consumed a small quantity of a household cleaning chemical a few days previously.

Bella was diagnosed with liver damage arising from exposure to the cleaning solution, which included toxic compounds damaging to the liver. Immediate action was undertaken, including supportive care to stabilize Bella's health, intravenous fluids to drain out the toxins, and drugs to boost liver function. With quick medication and attentive care, Bella eventually recovered, and her liver function improved over time.

Liver difficulties are widespread in dogs and may present as liver disease, toxicity, or failure, among other diseases. Understanding the symptoms and causes of liver disorders is critical for appropriate diagnosis and action. Through adequate veterinarian care, preventative steps to avoid toxin exposure, and supportive treatment, many liver disorders in dogs may be successfully cured or controlled, maintaining the health and well-being of our canine friends.

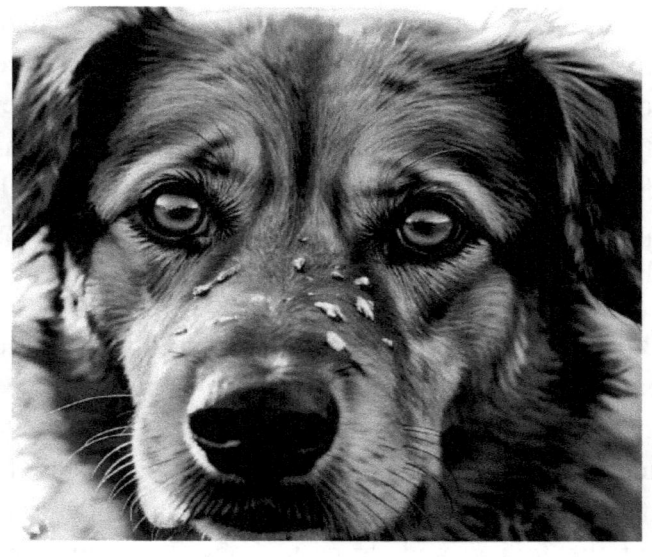

A photo of a dog showing signs of liver disease (e.g., yellowing of the eyes, skin lesions)

Signs and Symptoms of Liver Problems in Dogs (e.g., vomiting, diarrhea, lethargy)

The liver is a resilient organ, but when it encounters health issues, it often sends out distress signals through various signs and symptoms. Recognizing these indicators is vital for early detection and prompt intervention to prevent further complications. Here are some common signs and symptoms of liver problems in dogs:

1. **Jaundice (Yellowing of the Skin and Eyes)**: Jaundice is a classic sign of liver dysfunction in dogs. It occurs when there is an accumulation of bilirubin, a yellow pigment produced by the breakdown of red blood cells, in the bloodstream. Elevated levels of bilirubin can cause the skin, gums, and whites of the eyes to take on a yellowish hue. Jaundice may be accompanied by other symptoms such as dark urine, pale stools, and itchiness.

2. **Vomiting and Diarrhea**: Dogs with liver problems may experience gastrointestinal issues such as vomiting and diarrhea. These symptoms can occur due to impaired bile production, which affects the digestion and absorption of nutrients in the intestine. Vomiting and diarrhea may also result from toxins accumulating in the bloodstream due to

liver dysfunction, leading to gastrointestinal irritation and inflammation.

3. **Lethargy and Weakness**: Dogs with liver problems often exhibit lethargy, weakness, and reduced activity levels. The liver plays a vital role in metabolism and energy production, so when it's not functioning correctly, dogs may lack the energy and stamina to engage in their usual activities. Lethargy can be a subtle but important indicator of underlying liver issues and should not be overlooked.

4. **Decreased Appetite**: Loss of appetite, also known as anorexia, is a common symptom of liver problems in dogs. The liver plays a crucial role in regulating appetite and metabolism, so any disruption in its function can lead to changes in eating behavior. Dogs with liver issues may show disinterest in food, reluctance to eat, or even refusal to eat altogether, which can contribute to weight loss and nutritional deficiencies if left unaddressed.

5. **Abdominal Pain and Swelling**: Dogs with liver problems may experience abdominal discomfort and swelling due to inflammation or fluid accumulation in the abdominal cavity (ascites). Abdominal pain may manifest as restlessness, panting, reluctance to lie down, or guarding of the abdomen. Ascites, on the other

hand, can cause abdominal distension and a pot-bellied appearance in affected dogs.

Case Study: Identifying Liver Problems in Max

Max, a 6-year-old Golden Retriever, was brought to the veterinary clinic by his concerned owner, who noticed changes in his behavior and appearance. Max had become increasingly lethargic, his appetite had decreased, and his eyes appeared slightly yellow. Upon examination, Max's veterinarian detected jaundice, along with elevated liver enzymes on blood tests.

Further investigation revealed that Max had been exposed to a toxic plant in his backyard, which led to liver damage. Max also exhibited vomiting and diarrhea, which were attributed to gastrointestinal irritation caused by the toxins. Prompt intervention was initiated, including supportive care, fluid therapy, and specific treatments to support liver function.

Recognizing the signs and symptoms of liver problems in dogs is crucial for early detection and intervention. Jaundice, vomiting, diarrhea, lethargy, decreased appetite, and abdominal discomfort are common indicators of liver dysfunction. If you observe any of these signs in your dog, it's essential to seek veterinary attention promptly for proper diagnosis and treatment. Early intervention can help prevent further complications and improve the prognosis for dogs with liver issues.

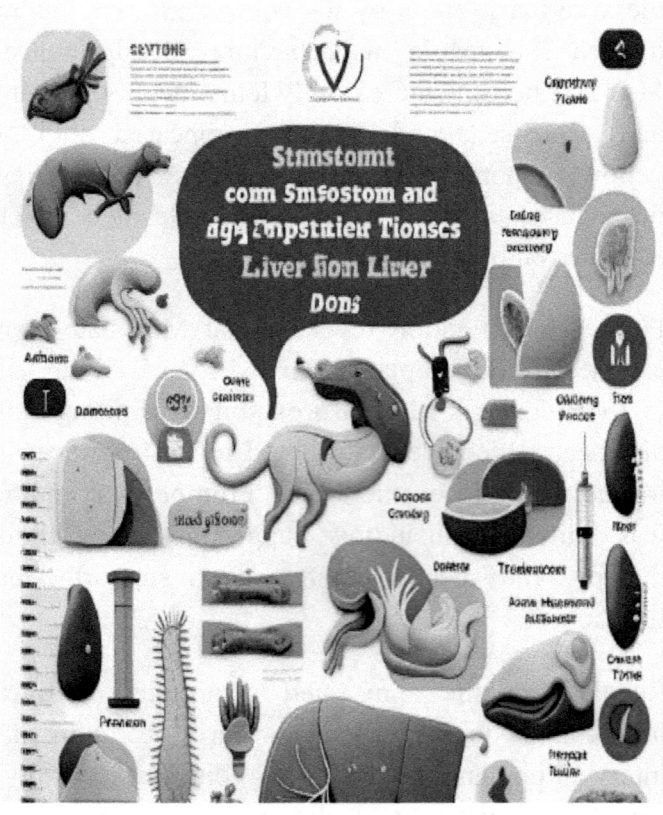

An infographic highlighting the common signs and symptoms of liver issues in dogs

CHAPTER 2:

NUTRITION AND LIVER HEALTH

The Role of Diet in Supporting Liver Function

Proper nutrition plays a crucial role in supporting liver health in dogs. A well-balanced diet that is tailored to the specific nutritional needs of dogs with liver issues can help alleviate symptoms, improve liver function, and promote overall well-being. Understanding the role of diet in supporting liver function is essential for managing liver conditions effectively.

1. **Protein Management**: Protein metabolism is closely linked to liver function, as the liver is responsible for processing and converting dietary proteins into usable forms. However, dogs with liver problems may have difficulty metabolizing protein, leading to an accumulation of ammonia and other toxic byproducts in the bloodstream. Therefore, it's important to manage protein intake carefully in dogs with liver issues. High-quality, easily digestible proteins such as lean meats (e.g., chicken, turkey) or eggs are recommended, while highly processed or low-quality proteins should be avoided. Additionally, feeding smaller, more frequent meals can help reduce the metabolic burden on the liver and improve protein utilization.

2. **Low Copper and Sodium Content**: Certain minerals like copper and sodium can exacerbate liver damage in dogs with liver issues. Excessive copper accumulation, in particular, is associated with certain breeds predisposed to copper storage diseases. Therefore, liver-friendly diets often contain reduced levels of copper and sodium to minimize the workload on the liver and prevent further damage. Choosing commercial dog foods specifically formulated for liver support or preparing homemade meals under the guidance of a veterinary nutritionist can ensure appropriate mineral content for dogs with liver problems.

3. **Essential Fatty Acids**: Omega-3 fatty acids, such as those found in fish oil, have anti-inflammatory properties and may help reduce inflammation in the liver. Incorporating sources of omega-3 fatty acids into the diet can benefit dogs with liver issues by promoting liver health and function. Fish oil supplements or diets rich in fatty fish like salmon or mackerel can provide these essential fatty acids. However, it's important to consult with a veterinarian to determine the appropriate dosage and ensure proper balance of omega-3 and omega-6 fatty acids in the diet.

4. **Antioxidants and Nutrient Support**: Antioxidants play a vital role in protecting liver cells from oxidative damage and promoting overall

liver health. Vitamins such as vitamin E and vitamin C, as well as other antioxidants like selenium and zinc, can help support liver function and reduce inflammation. Including foods rich in these nutrients, such as fruits, vegetables, and whole grains, in the diet can provide essential antioxidant support for dogs with liver issues. Additionally, supplementation with specific vitamins and minerals may be recommended based on individual nutritional requirements and the severity of the liver condition.

Case Study: Dietary Management of Canine Liver Disease

Meet Luna, a 9-year-old Beagle diagnosed with liver disease following abnormal liver enzyme levels on routine blood tests. Luna's veterinarian prescribed a liver-supportive diet tailored to her specific nutritional needs. The diet included a moderate amount of high-quality protein from lean meats, reduced copper and sodium content, and supplementation with omega-3 fatty acids and antioxidants.

Over time, Luna's symptoms improved, and follow-up blood tests showed a reduction in liver enzyme levels. Luna's liver-supportive diet, combined with veterinary care and medication, helped manage her liver disease and improve her overall quality of life.

Diet plays a crucial role in supporting liver function and managing liver conditions in dogs. A balanced diet that is tailored to the specific nutritional needs of dogs with liver issues can help alleviate symptoms, improve liver function, and promote overall well-being. By incorporating appropriate protein sources, managing mineral content, and providing essential fatty acids and antioxidants, pet owners can support their dogs' liver health and optimize their nutritional status. Consulting with a veterinarian or veterinary nutritionist is essential for developing an individualized dietary plan that meets the unique needs of each dog with liver issues.

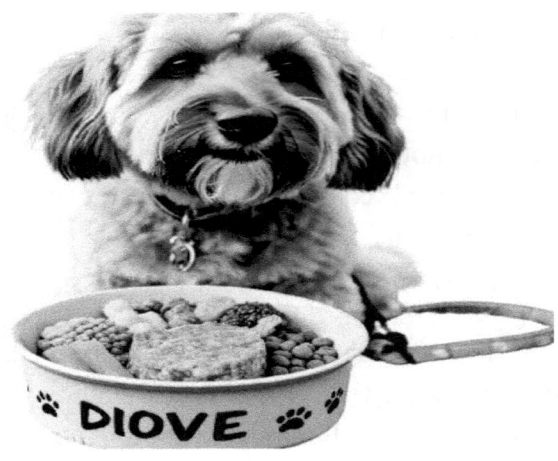

A photo of a healthy dog eating a balanced meal

Key Nutrients for Liver Health (e.g., vitamin E, omega-3 fatty acids, antioxidants)

Proper nutrition plays a vital role in supporting liver health in dogs, and certain key nutrients are particularly beneficial for promoting optimal liver function and preventing or managing liver issues. Understanding the importance of these nutrients and their specific roles in liver health is essential for selecting appropriate diets and supplements for dogs with liver conditions.

1. **Omega-3 Fatty Acids**: Omega-3 fatty acids, such as eicosapentaenoic acid (EPA) and docosahexaenoic acid (DHA), have anti-inflammatory properties and can help reduce inflammation in the liver. These fatty acids also support cell membrane integrity and function, which is important for liver health. Sources of omega-3 fatty acids include fish oil supplements, fatty fish (e.g., salmon, mackerel), and flaxseed oil. Incorporating omega-3 fatty acids into the diet can help support liver function and reduce oxidative stress in dogs with liver issues.

2. **Vitamin E**: Vitamin E is a powerful antioxidant that helps protect liver cells from oxidative damage caused by free radicals. It also plays a role in immune function and overall health.

Dogs with liver issues may benefit from supplementation with vitamin E to support liver function and reduce inflammation. Good dietary sources of vitamin E include nuts, seeds, and vegetable oils. However, supplementation should be done under the guidance of a veterinarian to ensure an appropriate dosage and avoid potential toxicity.

3. **Antioxidants**: Antioxidants are compounds that help neutralize harmful free radicals and reduce oxidative stress in the body, including the liver. Vitamins such as vitamin C and selenium, as well as phytonutrients like flavonoids and carotenoids, act as antioxidants and can help protect liver cells from damage. Fruits and vegetables, such as berries, citrus fruits, spinach, and carrots, are rich sources of antioxidants and can be included in a liver-supportive diet for dogs. Additionally, antioxidant supplements may be beneficial for dogs with liver issues, but dosage should be carefully monitored to prevent adverse effects.

4. **B Vitamins**: B vitamins play essential roles in liver metabolism and function, particularly in the metabolism of carbohydrates, fats, and proteins. Vitamins such as B6, B12, and folate are involved in processes such as energy production, detoxification, and the synthesis of essential molecules in the liver. Dogs with liver issues may

have increased requirements for B vitamins, and supplementation or inclusion of B vitamin-rich foods in the diet can help support liver health. Good dietary sources of B vitamins include meat, fish, eggs, dairy products, and whole grains.

Case Study: Nutritional Support for Canine Liver Disease

Meet Bailey, a 5-year-old Labrador Retriever diagnosed with liver disease following persistent vomiting, lethargy, and jaundice. Bailey's veterinarian prescribed a comprehensive treatment plan that included a liver-supportive diet rich in omega-3 fatty acids, vitamin E, antioxidants, and B vitamins.

Bailey's diet consisted of high-quality protein sources such as lean chicken and turkey, supplemented with fish oil for omega-3 fatty acids and vitamin E. Bailey also received antioxidant-rich fruits and vegetables as treats, along with a B-complex vitamin supplement to support liver metabolism.

Over time, Bailey's symptoms improved, and follow-up blood tests showed a reduction in liver enzyme levels. Bailey's nutritional support plan, combined with veterinary care and medication, helped manage her liver disease and improve her overall quality of life.

Key nutrients play a critical role in supporting liver health in dogs, and incorporating these nutrients into the diet can help prevent or manage liver issues. Omega-3 fatty acids, vitamin E, antioxidants, and B vitamins are particularly beneficial for promoting optimal liver function and reducing oxidative stress. Pet owners should work closely with their veterinarian to develop a tailored nutrition plan that meets the specific needs of their dog with liver issues, ensuring optimal support for liver health and overall well-being.

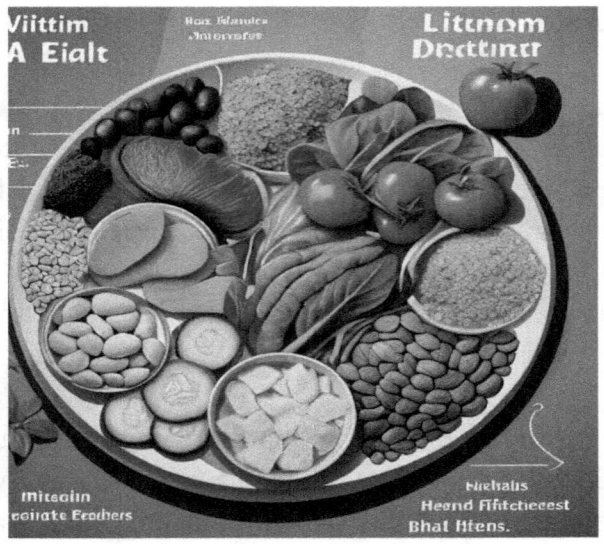

An illustration of the key nutrients and their benefits

How Hill's Prescription Diet l/d Supports Liver Health

Hill's Prescription Diet l/d (liver care) is specifically formulated to support liver health in dogs with liver conditions. This specialized diet provides targeted nutrition to help manage liver disease, reduce symptoms, and improve overall well-being. Let's explore how Hill's Prescription Diet l/d supports liver health:

1. **Reduced Protein Content**: Hill's Prescription Diet l/d contains a controlled amount of high-quality protein to support liver function without overloading the liver. Excessive protein intake can put strain on the liver, especially in dogs with liver conditions. By providing a balanced amount of protein, Hill's l/d helps minimize the metabolic burden on the liver and supports protein metabolism without exacerbating liver damage.

2. **High-Quality Protein Sources**: The protein sources in Hill's Prescription Diet l/d are carefully selected for their high digestibility and bioavailability. Ingredients such as chicken meal, pork fat, and egg products provide essential amino acids and nutrients necessary for maintaining muscle mass and supporting overall health in dogs with liver issues. These high-quality protein sources

are easily digestible and help meet the nutritional needs of dogs with compromised liver function.

3. **Reduced Copper and Sodium Levels**: Copper accumulation in the liver can contribute to liver damage in certain breeds predisposed to copper storage diseases. Hill's Prescription Diet l/d contains reduced levels of copper to help minimize the risk of copper-related liver issues. Additionally, the diet is formulated with controlled sodium levels to support fluid balance and reduce the workload on the liver, particularly in dogs with ascites (fluid accumulation in the abdomen).

4. **Added Antioxidants**: Antioxidants play a crucial role in protecting liver cells from oxidative damage and reducing inflammation. Hill's Prescription Diet l/d is enriched with antioxidants such as vitamin E and beta-carotene to help support liver health and function. These antioxidants help neutralize harmful free radicals, reduce oxidative stress, and promote the regeneration of healthy liver tissue in dogs with liver conditions.

5. **Omega-3 Fatty Acids**: Omega-3 fatty acids, such as EPA and DHA, have anti-inflammatory properties and can help reduce inflammation in the liver. Hill's Prescription Diet l/d contains added fish oil, a rich source of omega-3 fatty acids, to support

liver health and minimize inflammation. These fatty acids help maintain cell membrane integrity, support immune function, and contribute to overall liver function in dogs with liver issues.

Case Study: Efficacy of Hill's Prescription Diet l/d

Consider the case of Buddy, a 10-year-old Shih Tzu diagnosed with chronic liver disease characterized by elevated liver enzymes and jaundice. Buddy's veterinarian recommended Hill's Prescription Diet l/d as part of his treatment plan to support his liver health.

After several weeks on Hill's l/d, Buddy's symptoms began to improve. His jaundice faded, and follow-up blood tests showed a significant reduction in liver enzyme levels. Buddy's owner noticed an increase in his energy levels and appetite, indicating an improvement in his overall well-being.

Buddy continued to thrive on Hill's Prescription Diet l/d, and regular monitoring showed sustained improvement in his liver function. The targeted nutrition provided by Hill's l/d played a crucial role in managing Buddy's liver disease and enhancing his quality of life.

Hill's Prescription Diet l/d is specially formulated to support liver health in dogs with liver conditions. By providing controlled levels of high-quality protein, reduced copper and sodium content, added antioxidants, and omega-3 fatty acids, this specialized diet helps manage liver disease, reduce inflammation, and promote overall well-being in dogs with liver issues. With proper veterinary guidance, Hill's Prescription Diet l/d can be an effective component of a comprehensive treatment plan for dogs with liver conditions, helping them lead healthier and happier lives.

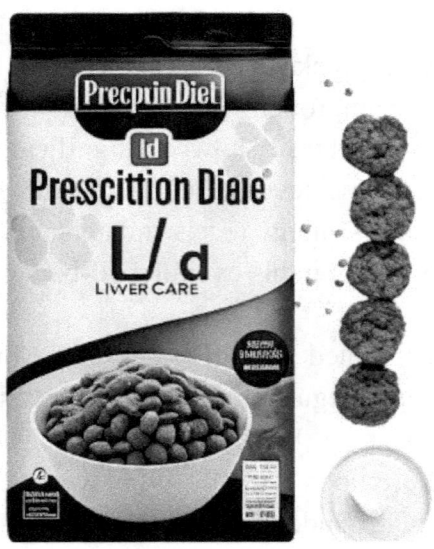

Picture: A product photo of Prescription Diet l/d Liver Care Dog Food

CHAPTER 3:
HILL'S PRESCRIPTION DIET L/D LIVER CARE DOG FOOD

Overview of the Product and its Formulation

Hill's Prescription Diet l/d (liver care) is a specialized dog food formulated to support liver health in dogs with liver conditions. This unique diet provides targeted nutrition to help manage liver disease, reduce symptoms, and improve overall well-being. Let's delve into the overview of Hill's Prescription Diet l/d and its formulation:

1. **Purpose and Target Audience**: Hill's Prescription Diet l/d is specifically designed for dogs with liver issues, including liver disease, hepatitis, hepatic lipidosis, and other liver-related conditions. It is formulated to provide nutritional support to dogs with compromised liver function, helping to alleviate symptoms, support liver regeneration, and improve overall quality of life. Hill's l/d is available by prescription and is recommended for use under the guidance of a veterinarian.

2. **Key Features and Benefits**:
    - **Controlled Protein Content**: Hill's l/d contains a controlled amount of high-quality protein to support liver function without overloading the liver. The carefully balanced protein content helps meet the nutritional needs of dogs while minimizing the metabolic burden on the liver.

    - **Reduced Copper and Sodium Levels**: The diet is formulated with reduced levels of copper and controlled sodium content to support liver health and minimize the risk of copper-related liver issues. Lowering copper intake helps prevent further liver damage in dogs predisposed to copper storage diseases.

    - **Added Antioxidants**: Hill's l/d is enriched with antioxidants such as vitamin E and beta-carotene to help protect liver cells from oxidative damage and reduce inflammation. These antioxidants help neutralize harmful free radicals, promote liver health, and support overall well-being in dogs with liver conditions.

    - **Omega-3 Fatty Acids**: The inclusion of omega-3 fatty acids from fish oil helps reduce inflammation in the liver and support liver function. EPA and DHA, the active components of omega-3 fatty acids, have anti-inflammatory properties and contribute to the overall health of dogs with liver issues.

3. **Ingredient Profile**: The formulation of Hill's Prescription Diet l/d includes high-quality ingredients that are selected for their nutritional value and digestibility. Key ingredients may include:

   - Chicken meal and pork fat as high-quality protein and fat sources.
   - Corn, barley, and rice as carbohydrate sources that are easily digestible and provide energy.
   - Beet pulp and flaxseed for added fiber, which supports digestive health and nutrient absorption.
   - Fish oil as a source of omega-3 fatty acids to reduce inflammation and support liver health.
   - Added vitamins, minerals, and amino acids to ensure a complete and balanced nutritional profile.

4. **Case Studies and Clinical Efficacy**: Hill's Prescription Diet l/d has been clinically proven to support liver health and improve clinical outcomes in dogs with liver conditions. Numerous case studies and veterinary testimonials attest to the efficacy of this specialized diet in managing liver disease, reducing symptoms, and enhancing the quality of life for dogs with liver issues. These real-life examples highlight the importance of

proper nutrition in supporting liver function and the positive impact of Hill's l/d on canine patients.

Hill's Prescription Diet l/d Liver Care Dog Food is a specialized diet formulated to support liver health in dogs with liver conditions. Its carefully balanced formulation, including controlled protein content, reduced copper and sodium levels, added antioxidants, and omega-3 fatty acids, provides targeted nutrition to help manage liver disease and improve overall well-being. With proper veterinary guidance, Hill's l/d can be an integral part of a comprehensive treatment plan for dogs with liver issues, helping them lead healthier and happier lives.

Key Ingredients and Their Benefits (e.g., high-quality protein, fiber, essential vitamins and minerals)

Hill's Prescription Diet l/d (liver care) dog food is formulated with carefully selected ingredients that provide targeted nutrition to support liver health in dogs with liver conditions. Each ingredient serves a specific purpose and offers unique benefits to help manage liver disease, reduce symptoms, and improve overall well-being. Let's explore the key ingredients of Hill's l/d and their benefits:

1. **High-Quality Protein Sources**:

   - **Chicken Meal**: Chicken meal is a concentrated source of protein derived from chicken meat. It provides essential amino acids necessary for muscle maintenance and overall health. The high-quality protein in chicken meal helps support lean muscle mass in dogs with liver issues while minimizing the metabolic burden on the liver.

   - **Pork Fat**: Pork fat is a highly digestible source of energy and essential fatty acids. It helps maintain healthy skin and coat, supports immune function, and provides palatability to the diet. Pork fat is a beneficial addition to Hill's l/d, as it contributes to the overall nutritional profile and taste appeal of the food.

2. **Digestible Carbohydrates**:

   - **Corn, Barley, and Rice**: These carbohydrate sources are easily digestible and provide a source of energy for dogs with liver conditions. They help maintain stable blood sugar levels and support overall metabolic function. Additionally, these grains contribute to the palatability and texture of the food, making it more appealing to dogs.

3. **Fiber-Rich Ingredients**:

   - **Beet Pulp**: Beet pulp is a source of soluble fiber that supports digestive health and promotes regular bowel movements. It helps maintain gut integrity, enhances nutrient absorption, and supports healthy digestion in dogs with liver issues. By including beet pulp in Hill's l/d, the diet promotes gastrointestinal health and ensures optimal nutrient utilization.

   - **Flaxseed**: Flaxseed is rich in soluble and insoluble fiber, as well as omega-3 fatty acids. It supports digestive health, reduces inflammation, and contributes to skin and coat health in dogs. Flaxseed is a valuable addition to Hill's l/d, as it provides essential nutrients that support overall well-being in dogs with liver conditions.

4. **Added Vitamins and Minerals**:

   - **Vitamin E**: Vitamin E is a powerful antioxidant that helps protect liver cells from oxidative damage caused by free radicals. It supports immune function, promotes skin and coat health, and contributes to overall well-being in dogs with liver issues. Vitamin E supplementation in Hill's l/d helps support liver health and reduce inflammation.

   - **B Vitamins**: B vitamins, including B6, B12, and folate, play essential roles in liver metabolism and function. They are involved in energy production, protein metabolism, and the synthesis of essential molecules in the liver. By including B vitamins in Hill's l/d, the diet supports liver health and ensures optimal nutrient metabolism in dogs with liver conditions.

Case Study: Efficacy of Key Ingredients in Hill's l/d

Casey, an 8-year-old Labrador Retriever, was diagnosed with chronic liver disease characterized by elevated liver enzymes and lethargy. Casey's veterinarian prescribed Hill's Prescription Diet l/d as part of his treatment plan to support his liver health.

After several weeks on Hill's l/d, Casey's symptoms began to improve. His energy levels increased, and follow-up blood tests showed a significant reduction in liver enzyme levels. Casey's owner noticed an improvement in his overall well-being, including a healthier coat and improved appetite.

Casey continued to thrive on Hill's Prescription Diet l/d, and regular monitoring showed sustained improvement in his liver function. The key ingredients in Hill's l/d, including high-quality protein sources, digestible carbohydrates, fiber-rich ingredients, and added vitamins and minerals, played a crucial role in managing Casey's liver disease and enhancing his quality of life.

Hill's Prescription Diet l/d Liver Care Dog Food is formulated with key ingredients that provide targeted nutrition to support liver health in dogs with liver conditions. High-quality protein sources, digestible carbohydrates, fiber-rich ingredients, and added vitamins and minerals offer unique benefits that help manage liver disease, reduce symptoms, and improve overall well-being. With proper veterinary guidance, Hill's l/d can be an effective component of a comprehensive treatment plan for dogs with liver issues, helping them lead healthier and happier lives.

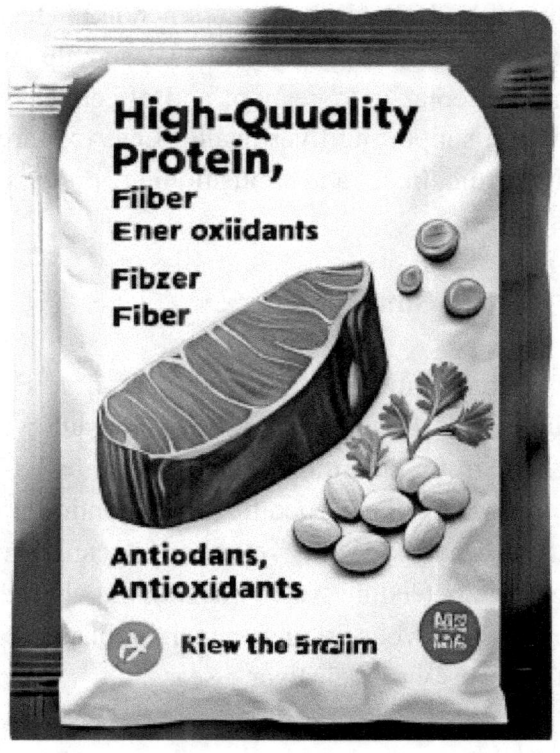

An illustration of the key ingredients (e.g., high-quality protein, fiber)

Feeding Guidelines and Transitioning to the Diet

Feeding guidelines and proper transitioning are crucial aspects of introducing Hill's Prescription Diet l/d (liver care) dog food to dogs with liver conditions. Following recommended feeding protocols and transitioning methods can help ensure optimal acceptance, digestion, and effectiveness of the diet in supporting liver health. Let's explore the feeding guidelines and transitioning process for Hill's l/d:

1. **Feeding Guidelines**:

   - **Consultation with a Veterinarian**: Before starting Hill's l/d, it's essential to consult with a veterinarian to determine the appropriate feeding plan for your dog's specific liver condition and nutritional needs. Your veterinarian can provide personalized feeding recommendations based on factors such as your dog's age, weight, health status, and the severity of their liver disease.

   - **Recommended Feeding Amounts**: Hill's Prescription Diet l/d provides specific feeding guidelines based on your dog's weight and nutritional requirements. It's important to follow these recommendations carefully to ensure your dog receives the appropriate amount of food each day.

Feeding too little or too much can impact your dog's health and may affect the effectiveness of the diet in managing liver issues.

- **Meal Frequency**: Dogs with liver conditions may benefit from smaller, more frequent meals throughout the day to help reduce the metabolic burden on the liver and support digestion. Dividing the daily recommended feeding amount into two or three meals can help maintain stable blood sugar levels and prevent excessive strain on the liver.

- **Water Availability**: Ensure that fresh, clean water is always available for your dog, especially when feeding a specialized diet like Hill's l/d. Proper hydration is essential for supporting liver function, promoting digestion, and maintaining overall health in dogs with liver conditions.

2. **Transitioning to Hill's l/d**:

- **Gradual Transition**: When transitioning to Hill's Prescription Diet l/d, it's important to introduce the new food gradually over a period of 7-10 days to avoid gastrointestinal upset. Start by mixing a small amount of Hill's l/d with your dog's current food, gradually increasing the proportion of

Hill's l/d while decreasing the amount of the old food each day.

- **Monitoring for Digestive Upset**: Keep a close eye on your dog's digestion and overall well-being during the transition period. Watch for signs of digestive upset such as vomiting, diarrhea, or changes in appetite. If your dog experiences any adverse reactions, slow down the transition process or consult with your veterinarian for guidance.

- **Patience and Persistence**: Some dogs may take longer to adjust to a new diet, especially if they have been eating the same food for an extended period. Be patient and persistent during the transition process, and provide encouragement and positive reinforcement to help your dog adapt to the new food. In most cases, dogs will gradually accept and enjoy Hill's l/d as their primary diet for supporting liver health.

Case Study: Successful Transition to Hill's l/d

Sammy, a 6-year-old Cocker Spaniel, was diagnosed with liver disease and prescribed Hill's Prescription Diet l/d by his veterinarian. Sammy's owner followed the recommended feeding guidelines and transitioned him to Hill's l/d over a period of 10 days.

During the transition, Sammy's owner closely monitored his digestion and overall well-being. Sammy experienced mild loose stools initially, but his symptoms resolved within a few days as he adjusted to the new diet. By the end of the transition period, Sammy was happily eating Hill's l/d as his primary food, and his energy levels had improved significantly.

Regular check-ups with Sammy's veterinarian showed positive progress in his liver function, and he continued to thrive on Hill's l/d as part of his treatment plan. The successful transition to Hill's l/d played a crucial role in managing Sammy's liver disease and improving his quality of life.

Feeding guidelines and proper transitioning are essential considerations when introducing Hill's Prescription Diet l/d Liver Care Dog Food to dogs with liver conditions. Following recommended feeding amounts, meal frequency, and transitioning methods can help ensure optimal acceptance, digestion, and effectiveness of the diet in supporting liver health. With patience, persistence, and veterinary guidance, Hill's l/d can be an integral part of a comprehensive treatment plan for dogs with liver issues, helping them lead healthier and happier lives.

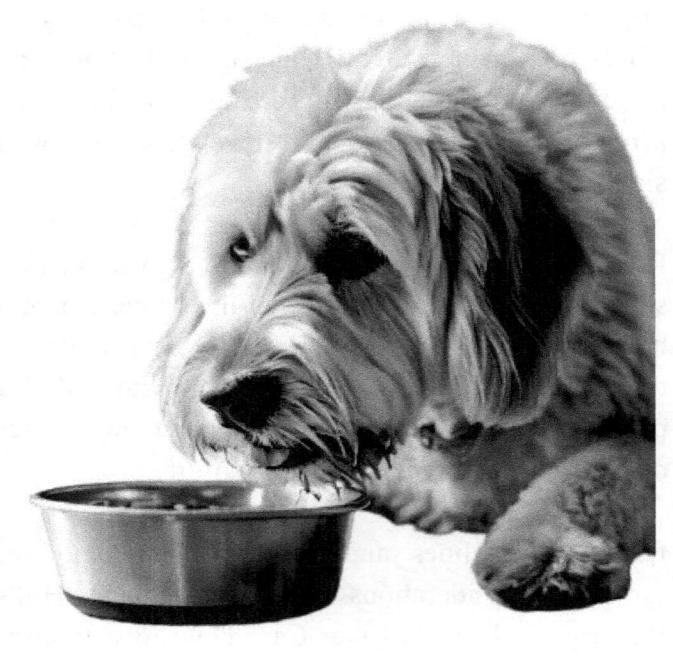

A photo of a dog eating a Prescription Diet l/d, and a gradual transition

CHAPTER 4:
MANAGING LIVER DISEASE IN DOGS

Diagnosis and Treatment Options (e.g., medication, surgery, dietary changes)

Diagnosing and treating liver disease in dogs requires a comprehensive approach that involves careful evaluation, diagnostic testing, and implementation of appropriate treatment modalities. From medication to surgery and dietary changes, each option plays a crucial role in managing liver disease and improving the prognosis for affected dogs. Let's explore the diagnosis and treatment options for liver disease in dogs:

1. **Diagnosis**:

   - **Physical Examination**: A thorough physical examination by a veterinarian is often the first step in diagnosing liver disease in dogs. Signs such as jaundice, abdominal pain, and palpable liver abnormalities may indicate liver dysfunction and prompt further investigation.

   - **Blood Tests**: Blood tests, including liver enzyme tests (e.g., ALT, AST, ALP), bile acid tests, and a complete blood count (CBC), can provide valuable information about liver function and identify abnormalities such as liver inflammation, impaired bile flow, or anemia.

- **Imaging Studies**: Imaging techniques such as ultrasound, X-rays, and MRI/CT scans may be used to evaluate the size, shape, and structure of the liver, as well as detect any masses, cysts, or abnormalities that may be contributing to liver disease.

- **Liver Biopsy**: In some cases, a liver biopsy may be necessary to obtain a tissue sample for microscopic examination. This procedure helps identify the underlying cause of liver disease, assess the severity of liver damage, and guide treatment decisions.

2. **Treatment Options**:

- **Medication**: Depending on the underlying cause and severity of liver disease, medication may be prescribed to manage symptoms, reduce inflammation, and support liver function. Medications such as antibiotics, anti-inflammatory drugs, antioxidants, and hepatoprotective agents may be used to address specific issues and improve liver health.

- **Dietary Changes**: Nutrition plays a crucial role in managing liver disease in dogs. Prescription diets such as Hill's Prescription Diet l/d Liver Care Dog Food are specifically formulated to support liver function and provide essential nutrients for dogs with liver conditions. These diets may contain controlled levels of protein, reduced copper and sodium content, added antioxidants, and omega-3 fatty acids to promote liver health and improve clinical outcomes.

- **Fluid Therapy**: Dogs with liver disease may experience dehydration, electrolyte imbalances, or fluid retention (ascites). Fluid therapy may be administered intravenously or subcutaneously to maintain hydration, correct electrolyte abnormalities, and manage fluid accumulation in the abdomen.

- **Surgery**: In some cases, surgical intervention may be necessary to address underlying causes of liver disease, such as liver tumors, cysts, or obstructed bile ducts. Surgical procedures such as liver lobectomy, bile duct reconstruction, or tumor removal may be performed by a veterinary surgeon to improve liver function and alleviate symptoms.

Case Study: Diagnosis and Treatment of Hepatic Lipidosis in Bella

Bella, a 7-year-old Persian cat, was presented to the veterinary clinic with signs of lethargy, vomiting, and jaundice. Blood tests revealed elevated liver enzymes and bile acids, indicating liver dysfunction. Ultrasound examination showed diffuse hepatic lipidosis (fatty liver disease), a common liver disorder in cats.

Bella was hospitalized for supportive care, including fluid therapy, nutritional support, and medication to manage her symptoms. The veterinarian prescribed Hill's Prescription Diet l/d Liver Care Cat Food to provide essential nutrients and support liver function. Bella responded well to treatment, and her symptoms gradually improved over several weeks of intensive care.

With continued monitoring and follow-up visits, Bella's liver function normalized, and she regained her energy and appetite. The combination of dietary management, medication, and supportive care played a crucial role in managing Bella's hepatic lipidosis and improving her overall quality of life.

Diagnosing and treating liver disease in dogs requires a multifaceted approach that encompasses thorough evaluation, diagnostic testing, and implementation of appropriate treatment modalities. From medication to surgery and dietary changes, each option plays a crucial role in managing liver disease and improving the prognosis for affected dogs. By working closely with a veterinarian and implementing a comprehensive treatment plan tailored to the individual needs of each dog, it's possible to effectively manage liver disease and optimize the quality of life for canine patients.

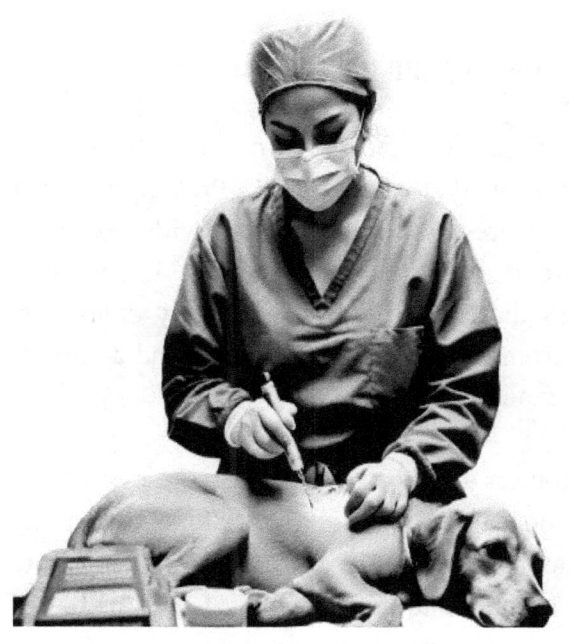

A photo of a veterinarian performing a liver biopsy or ultrasound on dog

Supporting Your Dog's Recovery and Ongoing Care

Supporting your dog's recovery from liver disease requires ongoing care, monitoring, and attention to their nutritional, medical, and emotional needs. After initial diagnosis and treatment, continued support is essential to promote healing, manage symptoms, and maintain overall well-being. Let's explore strategies for supporting your dog's recovery and ongoing care:

1. **Nutritional Support**:

   - **Tailored Diet**: Continue feeding a liver-supportive diet, such as Hill's Prescription Diet l/d Liver Care Dog Food, to provide essential nutrients and support liver function. Ensure that your dog's diet is well-balanced, easily digestible, and free from excess copper, sodium, and additives that may exacerbate liver issues.

   - **Monitor Appetite and Weight**: Keep track of your dog's appetite, eating habits, and body weight to ensure they are receiving adequate nutrition and maintaining a healthy weight. Loss of appetite or unintended weight loss may indicate underlying health issues that require veterinary attention.

2. **Medical Monitoring**:

   - **Regular Veterinary Check-ups**: Schedule regular follow-up appointments with your veterinarian to monitor your dog's liver function, assess response to treatment, and adjust management as needed. Blood tests, imaging studies, and physical examinations can help evaluate liver health and detect any changes or complications early on.

   - **Medication Management**: Administer any prescribed medications as directed by your veterinarian and monitor your dog for any adverse reactions or side effects. Communicate regularly with your veterinarian about your dog's response to treatment and any concerns you may have.

3. **Environmental Management**:

   - **Reduce Toxins and Chemical Exposures**: Minimize your dog's exposure to toxins, chemicals, and environmental pollutants that may contribute to liver damage. Keep household cleaning products, pesticides, and medications out of reach, and avoid exposing your dog to harmful substances in the environment.

- **Provide a Comfortable Environment**: Create a safe, comfortable environment for your dog to rest and recover. Ensure access to fresh water, a comfortable bed, and a quiet space away from noise and stressors. Environmental enrichment, such as interactive toys and mental stimulation, can also promote overall well-being during recovery.

4. **Emotional Support**:

  - **Provide Affection and Attention**: Offer plenty of love, affection, and attention to your dog during their recovery period. Spend quality time together, engage in gentle activities, and provide reassurance and comfort to help reduce stress and promote emotional well-being.

  - **Monitor Behavior Changes**: Pay attention to your dog's behavior and mood, and watch for signs of stress, anxiety, or depression. Changes in behavior, such as lethargy, aggression, or withdrawal, may indicate emotional distress and should be addressed with patience and understanding.

Case Study: Supporting Max's Recovery from Liver Disease

Max, a 4-year-old Golden Retriever, was diagnosed with liver disease following episodes of vomiting, diarrhea, and lethargy. After a thorough evaluation and diagnostic testing, Max's veterinarian prescribed a treatment plan that included medication, dietary changes, and ongoing monitoring.

Max's owner diligently followed the recommended feeding guidelines and transitioned him to Hill's Prescription Diet l/d Liver Care Dog Food to support his liver health. Regular check-ups with the veterinarian showed gradual improvement in Max's liver function, and his symptoms began to resolve over time.

In addition to medical management, Max's owner provided a supportive environment at home, ensuring he had access to plenty of water, rest, and affection. They monitored Max's appetite, behavior, and weight closely and communicated regularly with the veterinarian about his progress.

With dedicated care and ongoing support, Max made a full recovery from liver disease, and his quality of life improved significantly. By working closely with their veterinarian and providing comprehensive care, Max's owner played a vital role in supporting his recovery and ensuring his long-term well-being.

Supporting your dog's recovery from liver disease requires a holistic approach that encompasses nutritional support, medical monitoring, environmental management, and emotional support. By following recommended guidelines, providing attentive care, and working closely with your veterinarian, you can help your dog recover from liver disease and maintain a happy, healthy life. Remember to prioritize your dog's well-being and advocate for their needs throughout the recovery process, ensuring they receive the best possible care and support.

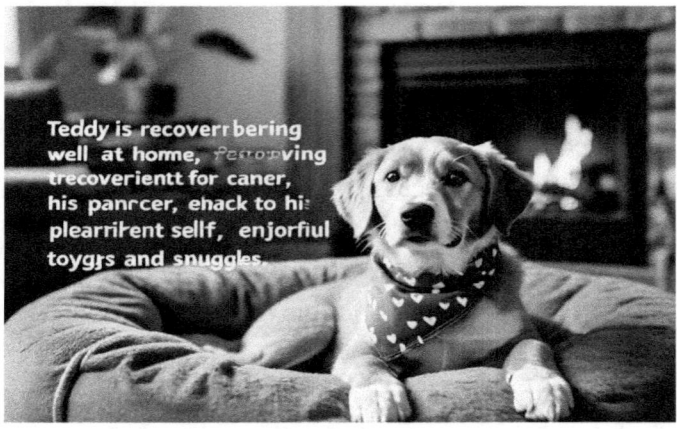

A photo of a dog recovering at home

Monitoring Progress and Adjusting the Diet as Needed

Monitoring your dog's progress and adjusting their diet as needed are essential components of managing liver disease effectively. Regular assessment of liver function, symptoms, and nutritional status allows for timely intervention and optimization of dietary management to support your dog's recovery and overall well-being. Let's explore strategies for monitoring progress and adjusting the diet as needed:

1. **Regular Veterinary Check-ups**:

    - **Liver Function Tests**: Schedule regular follow-up appointments with your veterinarian to monitor your dog's liver function through blood tests, including liver enzyme tests (e.g., ALT, AST, ALP) and bile acid tests. These tests provide valuable information about liver health and help assess response to treatment.

    - **Physical Examinations**: During veterinary check-ups, your veterinarian will conduct physical examinations to assess your dog's overall health and detect any changes in liver size, texture, or palpable abnormalities. Regular examinations allow for early detection of complications and adjustment of treatment plans as needed.

2. **Symptom Monitoring**:

   - **Observation of Clinical Signs**: Monitor your dog for any changes in symptoms associated with liver disease, such as vomiting, diarrhea, lethargy, jaundice, or changes in appetite and behavior. Keep a journal or log of your dog's symptoms, including their severity and frequency, to track progress over time.

   - **Communication with Your Veterinarian**: Report any changes or concerns about your dog's symptoms to your veterinarian promptly. Open communication allows for timely intervention and adjustment of treatment plans to address emerging issues and ensure optimal management of liver disease.

3. **Nutritional Assessment**:

   - **Body Condition Scoring**: Assess your dog's body condition regularly to ensure they are maintaining a healthy weight and body condition. Use a body condition scoring system recommended by your veterinarian to evaluate your dog's body composition and adjust feeding amounts accordingly.

- **Nutritional Consultation**: Consult with your veterinarian or a veterinary nutritionist to evaluate your dog's nutritional needs and ensure they are receiving adequate nutrition to support their liver health. Discuss any concerns or questions you may have about your dog's diet and make adjustments as needed based on their individual requirements.

4. **Dietary Adjustments**:

   - **Response to Treatment**: Evaluate your dog's response to dietary management and treatment for liver disease. If symptoms improve, liver enzyme levels normalize, and overall health improves, continue feeding the liver-supportive diet as recommended by your veterinarian.

   - **Reassessment and Modification**: If your dog's condition does not improve or worsens despite dietary management, discuss potential modifications to their diet with your veterinarian. Adjustments may include changes in protein content, addition of supplements, or exploration of alternative therapeutic diets based on your dog's specific needs.

Case Study: Adjusting Bailey's Diet for Optimal Liver Health

Bailey, a 9-year-old Beagle, was diagnosed with liver disease and prescribed Hill's Prescription Diet l/d Liver Care Dog Food by her veterinarian. Initially, Bailey's symptoms improved, and her liver enzyme levels decreased with dietary management.

However, after several months, Bailey's symptoms returned, and her liver enzyme levels began to rise again. Concerned about her lack of progress, Bailey's owner consulted with her veterinarian to reassess her treatment plan.

After further evaluation, Bailey's veterinarian recommended adjusting her diet to include additional nutritional support for her liver. Bailey was switched to a therapeutic diet formulated with higher levels of antioxidants, omega-3 fatty acids, and B vitamins to enhance liver function and reduce inflammation.

Over time, Bailey responded positively to the modified diet, and her symptoms improved once again. Regular monitoring showed sustained improvement in her liver function, indicating that the dietary adjustments were effective in supporting her recovery from liver disease.

Monitoring your dog's progress and adjusting their diet as needed are crucial aspects of managing liver disease effectively. Regular veterinary check-ups, symptom monitoring, nutritional assessment, and dietary adjustments allow for timely intervention and optimization of treatment plans to support your dog's recovery and overall well-being. By working closely with your veterinarian and providing comprehensive care, you can help your dog live a happy, healthy life despite liver disease.

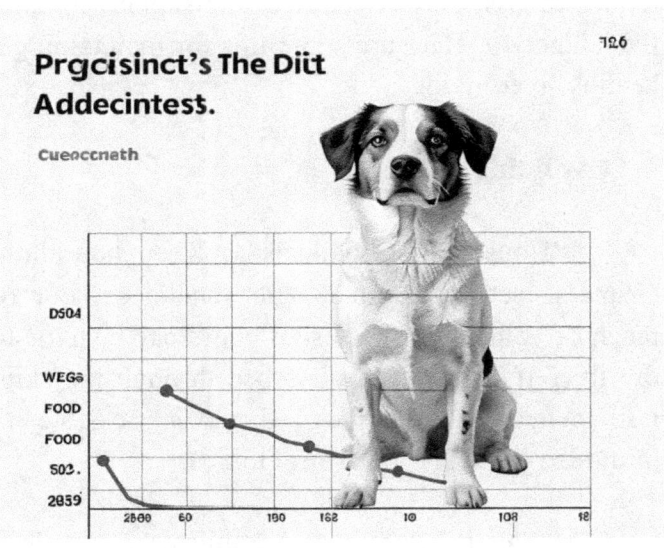

A graph or chart showing a dog's progress and adjustments to the diet

CHAPTER 5: PREVENTING LIVER ISSUES AND PROMOTING OVERALL HEALTH

Tips for Maintaining a Healthy Liver

Maintaining a healthy liver is essential for your dog's overall well-being and longevity. By implementing preventive measures and promoting liver health through lifestyle choices, you can reduce the risk of liver disease and support optimal liver function. Here are some tips for maintaining a healthy liver in dogs:

1. **Avoiding Toxins**:

   - **Household Chemicals**: Keep household cleaners, pesticides, and other chemicals out of reach of your dog. These substances can be toxic to the liver if ingested or absorbed through the skin. Use pet-safe alternatives whenever possible to minimize exposure to harmful toxins.

   - **Medication Safety**: Administer medications as directed by your veterinarian and store them securely away from pets. Certain medications, such as nonsteroidal anti-inflammatory drugs (NSAIDs), acetaminophen, and certain antibiotics, can cause liver damage if given inappropriately or at high doses.

- **Environmental Pollutants**: Minimize your dog's exposure to environmental pollutants such as cigarette smoke, air pollution, and industrial chemicals. These toxins can contribute to liver damage and increase the risk of liver disease over time.

2. **Providing a Balanced Diet**:

   - **Nutrient-Rich Diet**: Feed your dog a balanced, nutritious diet that supports liver health and overall well-being. Choose high-quality commercial diets or homemade recipes formulated to meet your dog's nutritional needs, including appropriate protein, fat, carbohydrates, vitamins, and minerals.

   - **Liver-Supportive Ingredients**: Incorporate liver-supportive ingredients into your dog's diet, such as antioxidants (e.g., vitamin E, selenium), omega-3 fatty acids (e.g., fish oil), and amino acids (e.g., taurine, methionine). These nutrients help protect liver cells from oxidative damage, reduce inflammation, and support liver function.

3. **Regular Exercise and Mental Stimulation**:

 - **Physical Activity**: Provide regular exercise and outdoor playtime to keep your dog active and maintain a healthy weight. Regular physical activity helps promote blood flow, metabolism, and overall organ function, including the liver.

 - **Mental Stimulation**: Engage your dog in mental stimulation activities such as puzzle toys, obedience training, and interactive games to keep their mind sharp and reduce stress. Mental stimulation promotes overall well-being and helps prevent boredom-related behaviors that may impact liver health.

4. **Routine Veterinary Care**:

 - **Annual Wellness Exams**: Schedule annual wellness exams with your veterinarian to monitor your dog's overall health and detect any potential issues early on. Regular check-ups allow for early detection and intervention, helping prevent the progression of liver disease and other health problems.

 - **Vaccinations and Parasite Control**: Stay up-to-date on vaccinations and parasite control to protect your dog from infectious diseases that can affect liver health. Preventing conditions such as canine hepatitis, leptospirosis, and heartworm disease helps maintain a healthy liver and immune system.

Case Study: Preventing Liver Issues in Luna

Luna, a 3-year-old Labrador Retriever, enjoyed exploring the outdoors with her owner and playing fetch in the park. Her owner made sure to provide a balanced diet consisting of high-quality commercial dog food supplemented with fresh fruits and vegetables rich in antioxidants.

Luna's owner also ensured that household chemicals and medications were stored safely out of reach, reducing the risk of accidental ingestion. Regular veterinary check-ups and vaccinations were scheduled to maintain Luna's overall health and prevent infectious diseases.

By incorporating preventive measures and promoting a healthy lifestyle, Luna's owner helped maintain her liver health and overall well-being. Luna continued to thrive, enjoying her active lifestyle and staying happy and healthy for years to come.

Maintaining a healthy liver in dogs requires proactive measures to prevent liver disease and promote optimal liver function. By avoiding toxins, providing a balanced diet, encouraging regular exercise and mental stimulation, and prioritizing routine veterinary care, you can help reduce the risk of liver issues and support your dog's overall health and longevity. Incorporate these tips into your dog's daily routine to ensure a happy, healthy life free from liver disease.

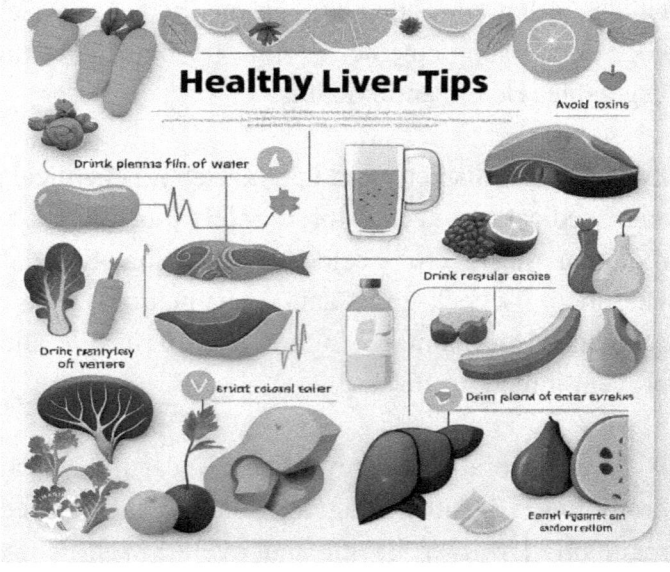

An infographic highlighting healthy liver tips (e.g., avoiding toxins, regular exercise)

The Importance of Regular Veterinary Check-Ups and Monitoring

Regular veterinary check-ups and monitoring play a crucial role in preventing liver issues and promoting overall health in dogs. These proactive measures allow veterinarians to assess your dog's liver function, detect early signs of liver disease, and implement preventive strategies to maintain optimal liver health. Let's delve into the importance of regular veterinary check-ups and monitoring:

1. **Early Detection of Liver Disease**:

   - **Liver Function Tests**: Routine blood tests, including liver enzyme tests (e.g., ALT, AST, ALP) and bile acid tests, help evaluate your dog's liver function and detect abnormalities that may indicate liver disease. Early detection allows for timely intervention and treatment, preventing the progression of liver issues and improving prognosis.

   - **Physical Examinations**: During veterinary check-ups, veterinarians perform physical examinations to assess your dog's overall health and detect any signs of liver disease, such as jaundice, abdominal pain, or palpable liver abnormalities. Regular examinations help identify subtle changes in your dog's condition that may require further evaluation.

2. **Monitoring Response to Treatment**:

   - **Treatment Follow-Up**: For dogs diagnosed with liver disease or at risk of developing liver issues, regular monitoring allows veterinarians to assess the response to treatment and make adjustments as needed. Monitoring liver enzyme levels, symptoms, and overall health status helps veterinarians evaluate the effectiveness of treatment and optimize management strategies.

   - **Dietary Management**: If your dog is prescribed a liver-supportive diet, such as Hill's Prescription Diet l/d Liver Care Dog Food, regular monitoring ensures that the diet is providing adequate nutritional support and meeting your dog's specific needs. Adjustments to the diet may be necessary based on your dog's response to treatment and changes in liver function over time.

3. **Preventive Health Care**:

   - **Vaccinations and Parasite Control**: Regular veterinary check-ups include vaccinations and parasite control measures to protect your dog from infectious diseases that can affect liver health.

Preventing conditions such as canine hepatitis, leptospirosis, and heartworm disease reduces the risk of liver damage and supports overall well-being.

   - **Dental Care**: Dental health is closely linked to liver health, as bacteria from periodontal disease can enter the bloodstream and affect the liver. Routine dental cleanings and oral examinations during veterinary check-ups help prevent dental issues and reduce the risk of secondary liver complications.

4. **Education and Guidance**:

   - **Client Education**: Veterinary check-ups provide an opportunity for pet owners to receive guidance and education on preventive care, nutrition, and lifestyle factors that impact liver health. Veterinarians can offer personalized recommendations based on your dog's age, breed, lifestyle, and health status to promote optimal liver function and overall well-being.

Case Study: Monitoring Molly's Liver Health

Molly, a 6-year-old Border Collie, was diagnosed with elevated liver enzymes during a routine veterinary check-up. Concerned about Molly's liver health, her veterinarian recommended further evaluation, including blood tests and imaging studies.

Following additional testing, Molly was diagnosed with liver disease, and a treatment plan was initiated, including medication and dietary management with Hill's Prescription Diet l/d Liver Care Dog Food. Molly's owner diligently followed the recommended monitoring schedule, scheduling regular veterinary check-ups to assess her liver function and response to treatment.

Over time, Molly's liver enzyme levels normalized, and her symptoms improved with ongoing management. Regular monitoring allowed Molly's veterinarian to evaluate her progress, make adjustments to her treatment plan as needed, and provide guidance on maintaining optimal liver health.

Regular veterinary check-ups and monitoring are essential components of preventive care for dogs, especially those at risk of liver issues. These proactive measures allow for early detection of liver disease, monitoring of treatment responses, implementation of preventive strategies, and client education on promoting optimal liver health. By prioritizing regular veterinary care, pet owners can help their dogs live long, healthy lives free from liver disease.

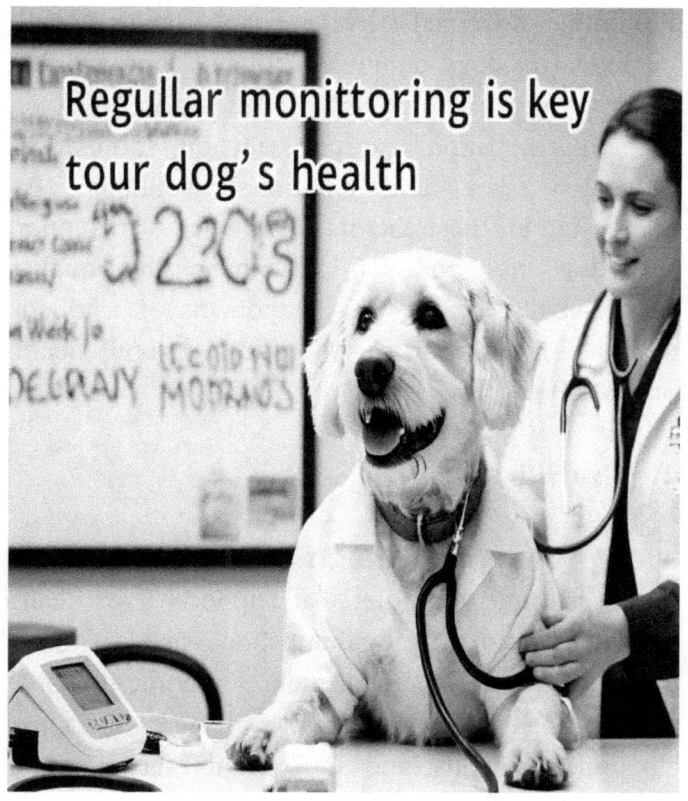

A photo of a dog at a veterinary check-up, with a caption about regular monitoring.

A Holistic Approach to Supporting Your Dog's Overall Health and Wellbeing

Promoting optimal liver health and overall wellbeing in dogs requires a holistic approach that encompasses various aspects of their lifestyle, including nutrition, exercise, mental stimulation, preventive care, and emotional wellbeing. By addressing all these factors, pet owners can support their dog's liver function and enhance their quality of life. Let's explore the components of a holistic approach to supporting your dog's overall health and wellbeing:

1. **Nutrition**:

   - **Balanced Diet**: Provide your dog with a balanced, nutritious diet that supports liver health and meets their individual nutritional needs. Choose high-quality commercial diets or home-prepared recipes formulated to provide essential nutrients, vitamins, minerals, and antioxidants necessary for optimal liver function.

   - **Liver-Supportive Ingredients**: Incorporate liver-supportive ingredients into your dog's diet, such as omega-3 fatty acids (found in fish oil), antioxidants (e.g., vitamin E, selenium), and amino acids (e.g., taurine, methionine). These nutrients help protect liver cells from oxidative damage, reduce inflammation, and support overall liver function.

2. **Exercise and Mental Stimulation**:

   - **Regular Exercise**: Provide your dog with regular opportunities for physical activity, such as walks, playtime, and interactive games. Regular exercise helps maintain a healthy weight, promotes circulation, and supports overall organ function, including the liver.

   - **Mental Stimulation**: Engage your dog in mentally stimulating activities to keep their mind sharp and prevent boredom-related behaviors. Offer puzzle toys, obedience training sessions, and interactive games to provide mental enrichment and reduce stress, which can impact liver health.

3. **Preventive Care**:

   - **Regular Veterinary Check-ups**: Schedule annual wellness exams with your veterinarian to monitor your dog's overall health and detect any potential issues early on. Routine blood tests, physical examinations, and dental check-ups allow for early detection of liver disease and other health problems.

- **Vaccinations and Parasite Control**: Stay up-to-date on vaccinations and parasite prevention measures to protect your dog from infectious diseases that can affect liver health. Preventing conditions such as canine hepatitis, leptospirosis, and heartworm disease reduces the risk of liver damage and supports overall wellbeing.

4. **Emotional Wellbeing**:

- **Positive Reinforcement**: Use positive reinforcement techniques to build a strong bond with your dog and promote positive behaviors. Offer praise, affection, and rewards for good behavior to enhance your dog's emotional wellbeing and reduce stress levels, which can impact liver function.

- **Routine and Stability**: Establish a predictable routine and provide a stable environment for your dog to thrive. Consistent feeding schedules, exercise routines, and social interactions help reduce anxiety and promote emotional stability, which is essential for overall wellbeing.

Case Study: Supporting Max's Holistic Wellbeing

Max, a 5-year-old German Shepherd, was adopted from a shelter by a loving family. Max's owners were committed to providing him with the best possible care and implemented a holistic approach to support his overall health and wellbeing.

They started by feeding Max a balanced diet consisting of high-quality commercial dog food supplemented with fresh fruits, vegetables, and omega-3 fatty acids. Max enjoyed regular walks, hikes, and playtime at the park, which provided both physical exercise and mental stimulation.

Max's owners scheduled annual wellness exams with their veterinarian, where Max received vaccinations, parasite control, and routine blood tests to monitor his liver function and overall health. They also enrolled Max in obedience training classes and provided plenty of opportunities for socialization with other dogs and people.

Through their holistic approach to Max's care, his owners observed improvements in his energy levels, coat condition, and overall demeanor. Max remained healthy, happy, and vibrant, enjoying a fulfilling life with his loving family.

A holistic approach to supporting your dog's overall health and wellbeing involves addressing multiple aspects of their lifestyle, including nutrition, exercise, mental stimulation, preventive care, and emotional wellbeing. By prioritizing these factors and providing comprehensive care, pet owners can promote optimal liver health and enhance their dog's quality of life. Remember to work closely with your veterinarian to develop a personalized care plan that meets your dog's individual needs and supports their holistic wellbeing.

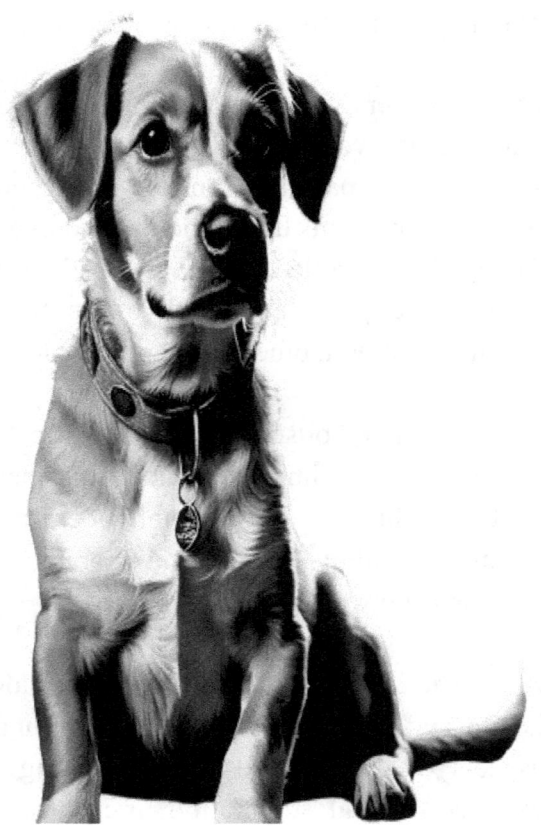

www.ingramcontent.com/pod-product-compliance
Lightning Source LLC
Chambersburg PA
CBHW050238230526
45470CB00005B/2015